I0494145

Hemp Seed Oil

The THC Free Healing Solution

By:

Ray Tokes

In our information obsessed societies, it's hard to comprehend a situation in which medical science isn't used to fully support something that helps people.

Yet, this is precisely the situation that cannabidiol and hemp oils currently find themselves in.

There is a vast wealth of information available about the various health benefits of hemp seed oil, but medical science has been slow to catch up.

While it is true that more research into the uses of hemp seed oil takes place every year, there is still a distinct sense of unease around this remarkable substance.

From a medical perspective, this apprehension is almost certainly due to its origin.

Hemp seed oil is derived from the cannabis plant, which also produces marijuana. However, hemp (neither the seeds nor the oil) does not contain THC, so it cannot get a person 'high.'

This means that, despite coming from the same place as marijuana, hemp seed oil couldn't be more different. For one thing, it has no value as a recreational drug. In some cases, it can induce feelings of relaxation and calm, but it doesn't have any psychotropic properties.

On the other hand, there is compelling evidence to suggest that it has the potential to alleviate the symptoms of everything from breast cancer to chronic migraines, diabetes, strokes, heart disease, joint pain, and more.

There is a huge amount of support for these claims, but most have not been fully peer reviewed or tested, due to the cultural unease around cannabis derivatives.

This is surely the next step though, because researchers and scientists are now starting to explore the impact that hemp seed oil has on the body.

The results, thus far, have been as impressive as expected. Hemp seed oil can be used to treat anxiety, relieve muscle pain, and maybe even delay cancer cells.

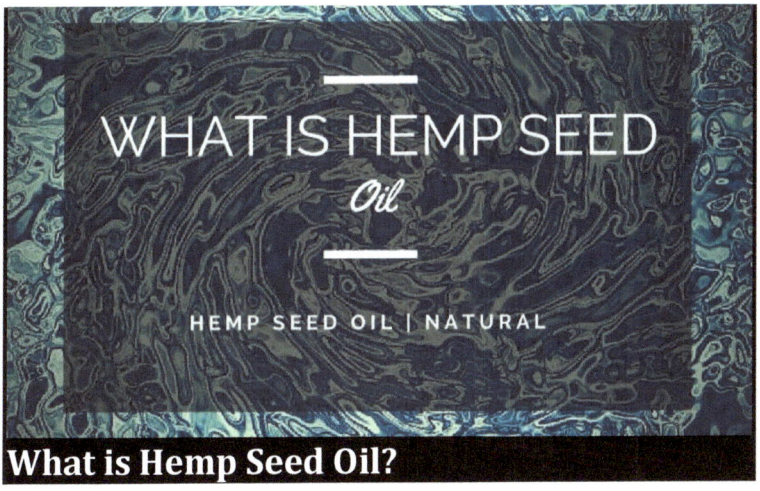

What is Hemp Seed Oil?

Most people know where hemp oil comes from, but fewer people know exactly what it is and what makes it so special.

This information is important, because it is used to distinguish hemp and hemp based products from those that contain THC.

In the US, the recreational use of THC is still illegal, so knowing the difference is advised. While marijuana (or weed) is made out of the flowers of the plant, hemp oil is extracted directly from its seeds.

It is filled with nutritional compounds that are great for the human body.

This is why hemp oil has been used medicinally and therapeutically for such a long time.

For example, hemp seed oil is packed with health boost omega 3 and omega 6 fatty acids.

They play an important part in keeping the brain functioning efficiently.

There is also evidence to suggest that it has antibacterial, antioxidant, antifungal, skin regenerative, antiviral, cardio-protective, and anti-inflammatory properties.

If used as a dietary supplement, it thickens hair, strengthens nails, alleviates acne, and calms the nerves.

As hemp seed oil is available in a wide variety of different forms, anybody can use it to boost their general health. Contrary to popular opinion, it does not have to be consumed raw; it can be added to salads, bought in flavored tinctures, and swallowed as dietary capsules.

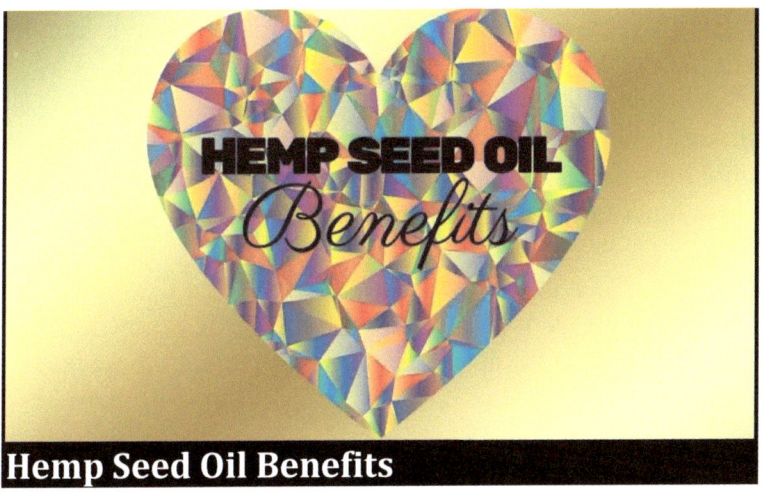

Hemp Seed Oil Benefits

Over the last decade, hemp seed oil has been linked to such a lengthy list of ailments that it's impossible to discuss them all.

It is believed, among other things, that hemp seed oil strengthens the immune system, regulates blood sugar, softens the skin, enhances the nervous system, lowers cholesterol, and improves the balance of bodily hormones.

It has also been linked to the disruption and delay of cancer cells.

It is likely that hemp seed oil has psychological benefits too, though it does not possess the same psychotropic qualities as marijuana.

A number of studies, though limited in their applicability and scope, have demonstrated a compelling link between anxiety disorders and treatment with hemp seed oil.

Hemp oil sprays and tinctures are particularly useful in this regard, because they can be activated almost instantly.

They only have to be sprayed or dropped into the mouth and their effects can be felt.

Given the established link between recreational marijuana smoking and paranoia, it may sound implausible to suggest that a derivative could be used to treat anxiety.

Yet, this is just one of the many features that distinguishes hemp seed oil from its THC filled relative. It is now known that the CBD in hemp oil actually counteracts the anxiety produced by THC.

Where one produces tension, the other dispels it.

For this reason, it is currently the focus of intense interest from scientists working on new anxiety medications.

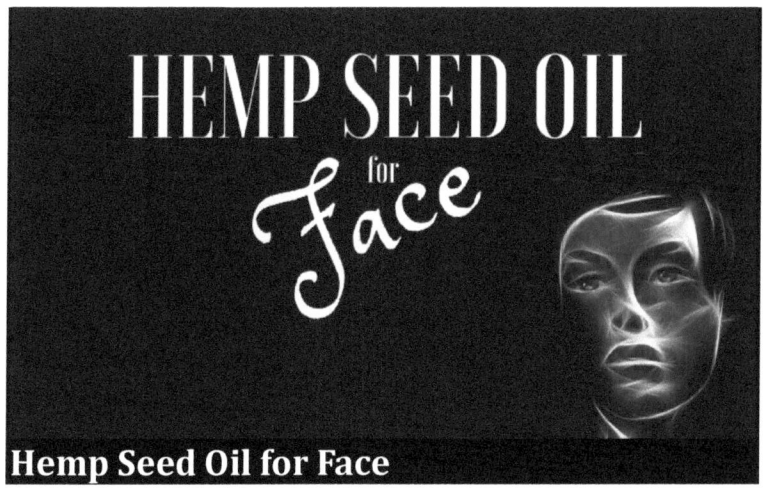

Hemp Seed Oil for Face

Hemp seed oil is a very nurturing substance for the skin and it is used, by many people, to treat chronic conditions like adult acne, eczema, psoriasis, and dermatitis.

It reduces moisture loss within the skin, so it is an effective solution for perpetual or seasonal dryness.

According to a Finnish study, hemp seed oil combats inflammation of the skin by providing the body with more omega 3 and omega 6 fatty acids.

After twenty weeks of treatment with hemp seed oil, the participants of the study saw a significant improvement in their symptoms; itching and discomfort was substantially reduced.

As most western diets lack these fatty acids, chronic skin conditions are common.

However, raw, unrefined hemp oil can be used to treat them either in the form of topical ointments or dietary capsules and sprays.

For all of these reasons, hemp seed oil is now regularly used in commercial cosmetics; everything from shaving creams to lip balms, sun screen, shampoo, and conditioner.

It acts as a natural moisturizer, so it helps the skin to feel smoother to the touch and it acts as a barrier against moisture loss.

Plus, it is rich in vitamin D, which plays a big part in calcium absorption rates and the nurturing of smooth, blemish free and hydrated skin.

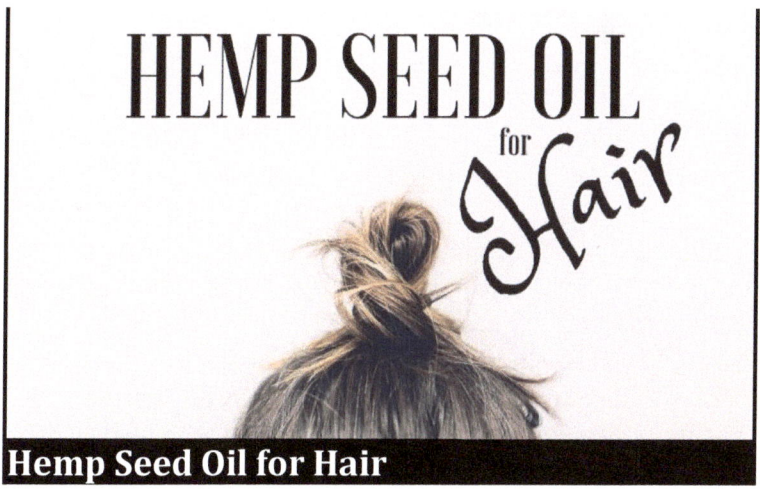

Hemp Seed Oil for Hair

It's not just the skin that hemp oil nourishes either, because it also has some rather wonderful benefits for the health of hair.

Those same fatty acids are just as effective at strengthening hair follicles and increasing shine and vitality.

Also, hemp seed oil is rich in vitamins and proteins, so it can be used to boost the health of all hair types; from the weakest, driest varieties to generally healthy tresses.

While the slightly nutty odor can be a little strange at first, it isn't unpleasant and applying hemp oil to the hair is easy.

It is available in either shampoo and conditioning products that contain hemp extracts, or raw oil can be applied directly to the hair and scalp.

This is the best way to take advantage of its benefits. Unrefined hemp seed oil can be bought in most good health food stores.

It will reduce water loss, keep the follicles soft, and support the scalp.

It is particularly effective when used in the winter months, as the cold weather can strip hair of its essential oils.

Hemp seed oil is a great replacement, but it should be bought in its purest form, unless it is being purchased as part of a 'natural' beauty product.

It doesn't have to be applied directly, however, because the benefits will also be felt if hemp seed oil is added to the diet as a supplement.

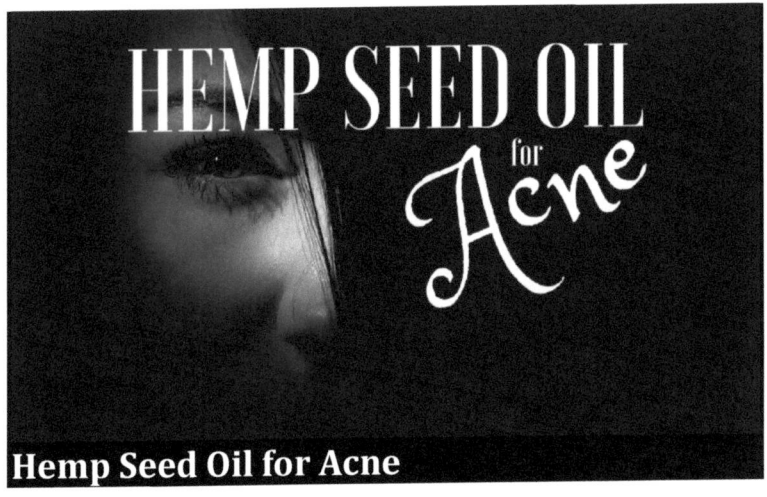

Hemp Seed Oil for Acne

The use of herbal remedies to treat acne is certainly not a new trend.

However, many of these treatments, though effective, cause the skin to 'purge' before they clear it up.

This means that the pores dispel all of the dirt and grime before clearing the skin and the user has to wait for the effects to kick in, so to speak.

Hemp seed oil is a little different, because it has a comedogenic rating of zero. This means that it treats the symptoms of acne without causing the skin to break out or the pores to become clogged up first.

As conditions like psoriasis and acne are often caused by a lack of omega 6 fatty acid in the diet, hemp oil makes sense as a topical or dietary treatment.

It hydrates the skin, increases the supply of oxygen, and reduces redness and inflammation.

As it is a natural plant derivative, within no known side effects for the skin, it is completely safe for use on the face and other areas of the body.

If all of this weren't enough, hemp seed oil also supports the skin when it comes to regulating the production of sebum.

Sebum is an interesting substance, because it can be both beneficial and detrimental for the skin.

It is designed to provide lubrication, but if there is a lack of linoleic acid in the diet, it becomes sticky and more prone to clogging up pores.

Fortunately, hemp seed oil contains around 60% linoleic acid.

For those with chronic acne or other skin problems, it can be consumed the form of dietary capsules, sprayed in the mouth in the form of a tincture, or even eaten in protein powders.

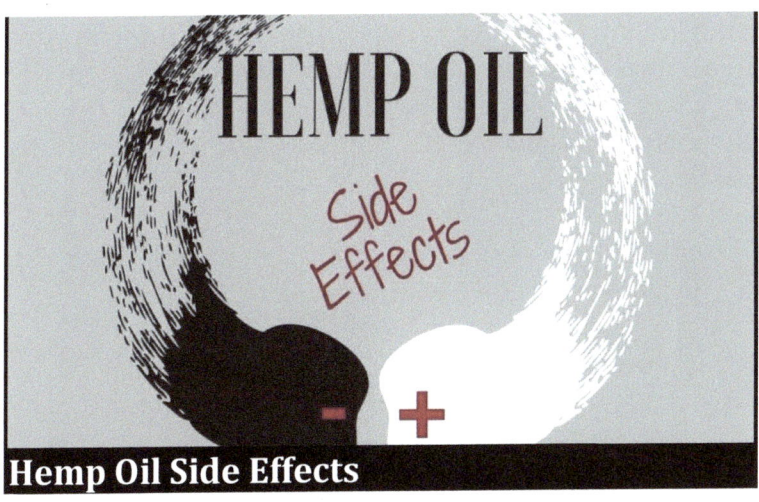

Hemp Oil Side Effects

When it comes to general side effects of using hemp oil for health, information is mostly vague.

There is some evidence to suggest that the substance has a number of minor side effects, for some people, but this has not been medically verified or tested.

For anybody planning to use hemp seed oil as a dietary supplement, it is important to review all of the available information first and come to a personal judgement.

Hemp seed oil is very rich in omega fatty acids, which are hugely beneficial for the body, but they shouldn't be ingested in overly large doses.

An overabundance of polyunsaturated fatty acids has been linked to conditions like cardiac dysfunction and vulnerability to bacterial infections.

So, users should always avoid consuming more hemp seed oil than is recommended by manufacturers and health food experts.

Furthermore, hemp seed oil should never be cooked at very high temperatures (above 121 degrees Fahrenheit).

Not only will this cause the oil to turn rancid, it also produces toxic peroxides.

For this reason, hemp seed oil should only ever be consumed raw or served with warm and cold dishes.

For a very small number of people, dietary hemp supplements can aggravate existing bowel conditions.

It is best to find a substitute supplement if chronic bowel problems are an existing condition.

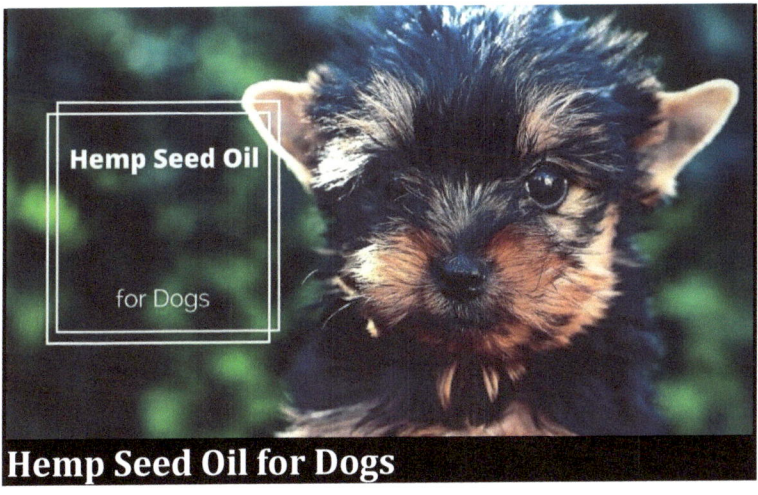

Hemp Seed Oil for Dogs

It is also possible to supplement canine diets with hemp seed oil, if the right products are used, in safe amounts.

In fact, most of the health benefits enjoyed by humans can also be enjoyed by dogs; for example, softer skin, shinier hair, a stronger immune system, and reduced inflammation and skin allergies.

As hemp seed oil has no psychotropic properties, it will not harm dogs or have a detrimental impact on their mood or personality.

However, there are a few things that need to be considered before a dog is given hemp seed oil. The first is that the substance should never be cooked. This will cause the oil to turn rancid and produce harmful toxins.

Therefore, if it is being added to pre-cooked dog food, it needs to be incorporated immediately before serving. One teaspoon per day is more than enough, even for large dogs; remember that too much hemp oil can be bad for the health.

If a canine diet is safely supplemented with hemp seed oil, it will improve the condition of the skin and fur, reduce the rate of shedding, encourage healthy organ function, and support the growth of the brain.

The only time that hemp oil is not suitable is when a dog is being fed a special protein packed diet. As hemp seed oil is also protein rich, combining it with a poultry heavy diet will lead to an imbalance of healthy fats and linoleic acid. In this case, flaxseed oil is the safest, healthiest alternative to hemp oil.

Contrary to popular belief, it doesn't have to be used as a vaping solution or tincture.

It also doesn't have to be sprayed directly into the mouth if there is discomfort or anxiety around doing so.

As an alternative, there are hemp seed oil capsules, protein powders, specially formulated supplements, and raw shelled (edible) seeds.

This level of variety makes it much easier for people who are unfamiliar with hemp seed oil to experiment with different products and find one that suits their routine and lifestyle.

It is certainly worth doing a little research into the respective benefits of each product, because they all cater for slightly different needs. For example, people with anxiety problems can use hemp seed oil to alleviate the symptoms.

With capsules, the effect is almost instant, which makes them the best option for this particular need.

The downside to this level of variety is that it can also make it quite hard to pick the right hemp seed oil product.

With so many options to choose from, the uninitiated can sometimes feel a little intimidated.

The best place to start for those who have never tried hemp seed oil before is with dietary capsules.

They are easy to take, because they work in much the same way as any other kind of supplement.

They are swallowed whole, once or twice a day, usually around mealtimes or in the morning and evening.

There are no serious side effects associated with the use of hemp seed oil, as long products are used correctly and according to guidance from the manufacturer.

One important thing to remember is that it should not be exposed to high temperatures.

Too much heat causes the polyunsaturated fatty acids to break down and the oil turns rancid.

It can be served, as a dressing on warm meals, but it should not be used for cooking.

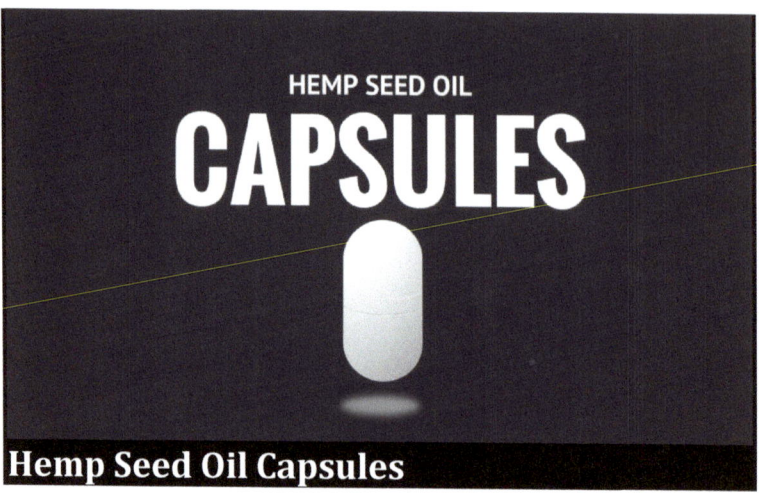

Hemp Seed Oil Capsules

One of the easiest ways to introduce hemp seed oil into the diet is with basic, supplementary capsules.

These are no different to things like the flaxseed oil or cod liver oil capsules found in most heath stores.

They are packaged in a soft glycerin shell, which makes takes away any discomfort when swallowing and helps them break down once they reach the digestive system.

Hemp seed oil capsules are the best option for those who are interested in boosting their overall health with the use of this supplement.

The hemp seed oil found in capsules is the same substance that is bought as raw oil or used in vaping tinctures.

However, some people don't like the taste, so capsules allow them to enjoy its benefits without experiencing the flavor too.

The taste of hemp seed oil can be an acquired one, but it isn't overly strong or overpowering.

It has a slightly nutty flavor, which actually makes it a great substitute for people who suffer with nut allergies.

The added advantage of supplementing with capsules, of course, is that they are discreet.

If there is any reticence or anxiety about being seen to ingest a cannabis derivative – though it is entirely legal – capsules allay these feelings.

Unless investigated at close quarters, they look just like any other kind of capsule based supplement.

It is also worth pointing out that consumption via tablets gives the user as much control as possible over what they are putting into their body.

Each capsule contains an identical amount of hemp seed oil, so there is no risk of unintentionally consuming more than recommended.

Taking a controlled volume, on each occasion, is helpful because it provides a more stable and predictable outcome.

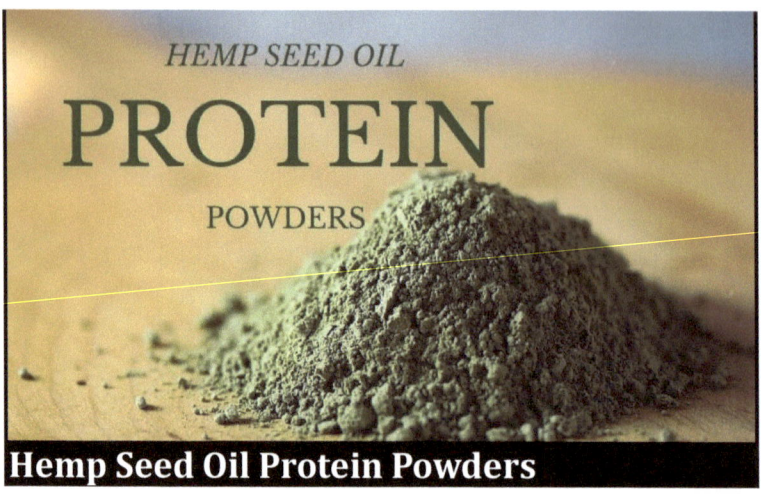

Hemp Seed Oil Protein Powders

The most common ways to consume hemp seed oil are in the form of tinctures, raw unrefined oils, and dietary capsules.

However, it is also possible to purchase hemp oil in the form of nutritious protein powders.

They are the recommended option for anybody who wants to eat their hemp seed oil in things like cakes and smoothies.

Protein powders are a little less sensitive to extreme heat than raw oil, but it is still important to exercise care and stick to low temperatures when cooking with this substance.

On average, there is around 15g of protein in every individual serving of hemp seed oil powder. This makes it a very nourishing addition to an already healthy and balanced lifestyle.

Vegetarians tend to find hemp oil protein powders really useful, because they are all natural and do not contain any animal fats and animal based ingredients.

They are also a popular choice among weightlifters and athletes, as they boost protein intake and contribute to the smooth functioning of joints and muscles.

Protein powders speed up the regeneration of lean body mass. In order to this, they increase the levels of branched amino acids.

Hemp seed oil is rich in these acids, so it is extremely effective when it comes to muscle repair.

It is also filled with cysteine and methionine and both of these compounds are needed to create essential enzymes.

The only downside to hemp seed oil powders is that they are designed to provide a sustained boost.

For this reason, they are probably not the best choice for people looking to see quick results.

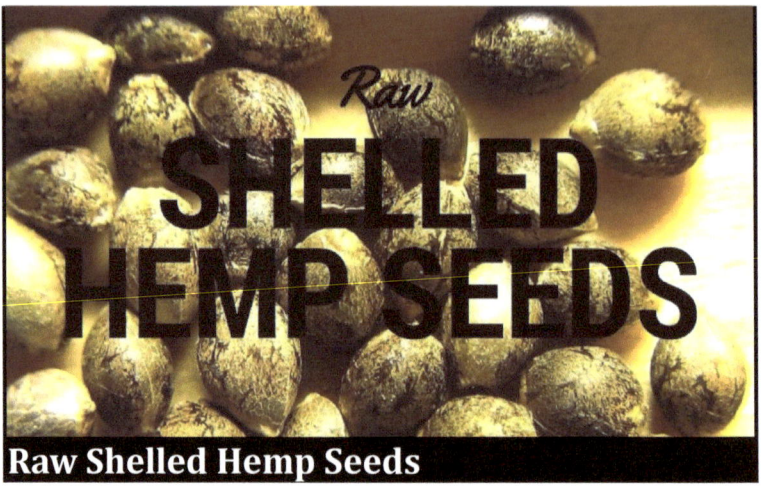

Raw Shelled Hemp Seeds

Hemp seed oil may also be ingested and added to the diet in the form of raw, shelled hemp seeds.

Once again, these are much like the sunflower seeds that are found in health food stores.

They can be eaten right out of the bag or container, but lots of people prefer to sprinkle them on salads or add them to smoothies.

Raw hemp seeds are another great way to enjoy the lasting health benefits of this nourishing substance.

In their pure, shelled form, they don't taste anywhere near as strong as raw oil, so they helpful for sensitive palettes.

Like raw oil, the seeds should not be exposed to high temperatures or cooked at high heats.

They will turn rancid and become unsafe for consumption. However, they are perfectly safe if eaten on top of warm salads or sprinkled on healthy foods like granola.

Raw hemp oil seeds contain large amounts of a substance called globulin edistin.

It is a simple protein with remarkable powders. It provides the body with everything that it needs to fight off infections and other kinds of sickness.

Crucially, the human body can't actually create its own globulin edistin.

It has to be acquired from foods that are rich in the compound.

Fortunately, hemp seed oil is one of these foods. In various different regions across the world (China, for example), raw hemp seeds have been eaten for a long time.

They have a nutty, warm flavor that some people really love and regularly enjoy in salads, soups, and fibre heavy cereals.

The amount of THC contained in hemp seeds is so small that it is not quantifiable. Eating the seeds cannot got a person 'high.'

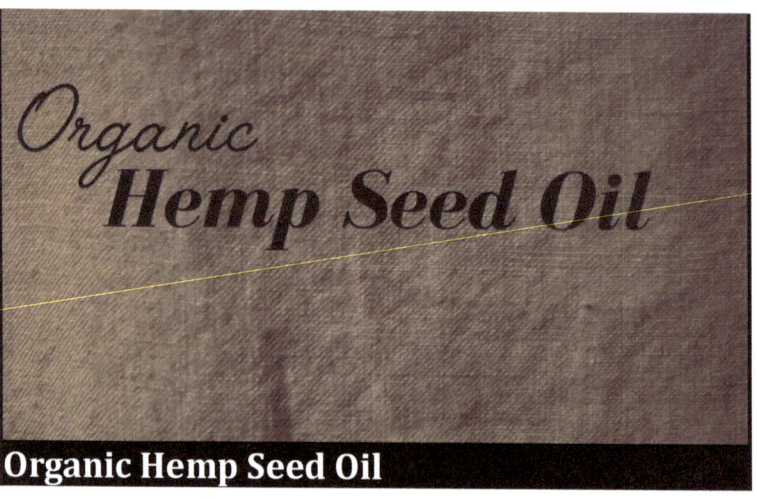

Organic Hemp Seed Oil

Lastly, there is organic hemp oil, in its purest form.

This is sold much like cooking oil would be, but it cannot be used in conjunction with high heat.

The best products are unrefined and cold pressed; they should be all natural, with very little manufacturing or processing after extraction.

Organic hemp seed oil can be drizzled over pizzas, salads, stir fries, pasta dishes, potatoes, and much more. It also makes a delicious dip for warm, crusty bread.

Alternatively, if the taste is not enjoyed, it can be disguised in soups, shakes, and smoothies.

Organic hemp oils need to be carefully stored, because if they are exposed to too much heat or sunlight, the nutritional value of the seeds will be compromised.

Ideally, hemp oil should be consumed within four months after opening. These requirements mean that it isn't always the most suitable choice for people looking for an occasional dietary supplement.

Capsules, [tinctures](), and protein powders all have a much longer shelf life. On the other hand, they are great for vegetarians.

They contain only natural compounds and absolutely no animal fats.

These products are full of omega fatty acids, fibre, and protein, all of which are needed by the body for regeneration, growth, repair, and fortification.

With no less than twenty essential amino acids, there are few dietary supplements as impressive as this on the market.

Organic hemp seed oil can be bought online and from many health food stores.

It is important to buy from a reputable dealer, with a trusted reputation for providing high quality products.

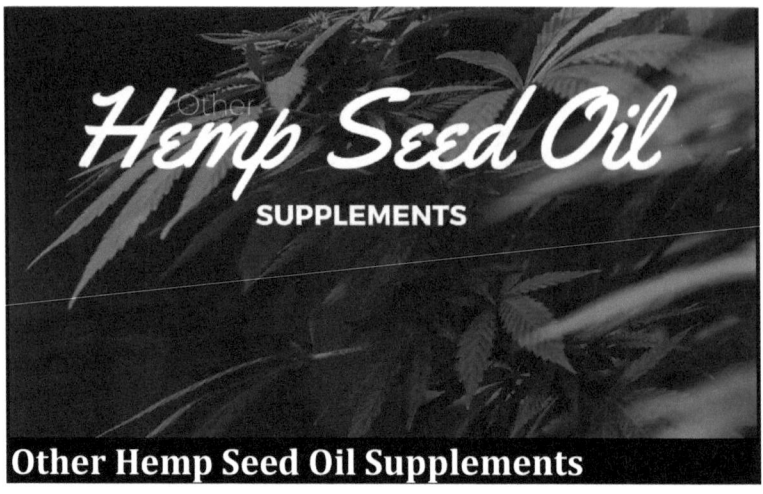

Other Hemp Seed Oil Supplements

For a fast acting boost, there are hemp seed oil sprays and tinctures.

These products work with the use of direct application. They are usually sprayed or dropped beneath the tongue, because this allows them to get to work quickly.

Tinctures and sprays are a popular form of dietary supplement. This is primarily because they are so easy to use. They are also pretty discreet. Like hemp seed oil capsules, they can be carried in the pocket or in a handbag.

It is important to point out that tinctures and sprays are not just faster than other forms of hemp seed oil, they are also more powerful.

They provide a stronger, less diluted hit, so they should only be considered once this is recognized and understood.

The good news is that spray bottles and tincture formulas are easy to monitor.

Each spray or drop contains an identical amount of hemp seed oil (and CBD), so it is rare to ingest more than recommended.

The downside is that there tends to be more intensity to the flavor.

For people who are not fond of the taste of hemp seed oil, capsules or powders are a better choice.

Some tinctures also contain alcohol, so do be aware of this when shopping.

If an alcohol free formula is desired, search specifically for all-natural products.

For people who dislike swallowing pills, sprays and tinctures offer an easy to use, no fuss alternative.

Important Things to Consider When Shopping

CBD hemp oil is a dietary and lifestyle supplement that is made out of industrial hemp.

It is legally available in all of the US states. The purchase of CBD oil does not require any kind of prescription or permit.

Nevertheless, caution should be taken when shopping for hemp seed oil products, as there is a wide variety of options available on the market.

The legislation associated with the production of hemp seed oil is still in its infancy, so consumers have a responsibility to be informed and aware.

From a cultural and social perspective, hemp is in a rather curious position.

It is distributed and sold widely, in a multitude of different forms, but its many medical benefits still lack peer reviewed testing.

It is broadly agreed that hemp seed oil is a safe substance.

There are few known side effects and the ones that we do know about only manifest themselves when hemp oil is consumed in extreme quantities.

However, this lack of firm scientific support means that a healthy degree of caution should be taken when using it.

This means following the instructions provided by the manufacturer at all times.

It also means storing hemp seed oil products in the recommended way, so that they do not turn rancid and produce toxic compounds.

Largely though, safe use just refers to common sense; use one hemp seed oil product at a time, avoid exposure to extreme temperatures, and enjoy it as part of a balanced lifestyle.

This last piece of advice is crucial, because there are no magic health supplements. They are only effective if incorporated into an already healthy diet and routine.

Source - http://cannabiscbdoil.org